END YOUR CONFUSION
ON
CARB DIET

Unveiling the myth and fact of carbohydrates

and the health impact on your body

SARAH BILLY

Table of Contents

Snack Recipes for Balanced Carb Meals 93

Chapter 1

Introduction

Understanding Carbohydrates

Carbohydrates are fundamental macronutrients crucial for sustaining the body's energy needs. Composed of carbon, hydrogen, and oxygen atoms, carbohydrates exist in various forms, with monosaccharides (single sugar molecules) and polysaccharides (complex sugar structures) being primary components.

Carbohydrates, often referred to as carbs, are a diverse group of compounds consisting of carbon, hydrogen, and oxygen. They can be classified into two main types: simple carbohydrates and complex carbohydrates.

Simple carbohydrates, found in fruits, honey, and processed foods, consist of easily digestible sugars like glucose and fructose. In contrast, complex carbohydrates, prevalent in whole grains, legumes, and vegetables, provide sustained energy due to their longer sugar chains.

The body relies on carbohydrates as a primary energy source. When consumed, they are broken down into glucose, which fuels cellular functions. Excess glucose is stored in the liver and muscles as glycogen, serving as a reserve for energy demands.

Dietary sources of carbohydrates include whole grains like brown rice and oats, nutrient-rich fruits and vegetables, and protein-packed legumes such as beans and lentils. Fiber, a complex carbohydrate found in these foods, aids digestion and promotes a feeling of fullness.

Understanding the glycemic index helps regulate blood sugar levels. Choosing complex carbohydrates, coupled with fiber and protein, mitigates rapid spikes in blood sugar, promoting sustained energy release.

Individual carbohydrate needs vary based on factors like age, activity level, and health status. Balancing carbohydrate intake with proteins and fats ensures a well-rounded diet.

While carbohydrates are essential, the quality of their sources matters. Opting for whole, unprocessed carbohydrates supports overall health, while excessive consumption of refined options may contribute to weight gain and metabolic issues.

Common Misconceptions

Carbohydrates often face misconceptions that can impact dietary choices. It's essential to debunk these myths for a more informed approach to nutrition.

Carbs are All the Same: A prevalent myth assumes that all carbohydrates are equal. In reality, there are simple carbohydrates (found in sugary snacks) and complex carbohydrates (present in whole grains and vegetables). Opting for complex carbs provides sustained energy and essential nutrients.

Carbs Lead to Weight Gain: Another misconception suggests that consuming carbohydrates inevitably leads to weight gain. The truth is that excess calories, regardless of the macronutrient, contribute to weight gain. Balancing carb intake with overall calorie consumption and choosing whole, nutrient-dense options is key.

Low-Carb Diets are the Only Solution: Some believe that the only way to achieve health and weight loss is through a low-carb diet. While reducing refined carbs can be beneficial, eliminating carbohydrates is unnecessary and can deprive the body of essential nutrients.

Carbs are Unhealthy: Carbohydrates are a vital energy source and offer various health benefits when chosen wisely. Whole grains, fruits, and vegetables provide essential vitamins, minerals, and fiber necessary for overall well-being.

Carbs Cause Diabetes: Carbohydrates alone do not cause diabetes. Type 2 diabetes is influenced by various factors, including genetics, lifestyle, and overall diet. Consuming a balanced diet and managing portion sizes play a crucial role in diabetes prevention.

Avoiding Carbs Enhances Performance: Athletes often fear that consuming carbs hinders performance. In reality, carbohydrates are a primary energy source during physical activity, and adequate intake is crucial for endurance and stamina.

Chapter 2

The Role of Carbs in Your Diet

Importance of Carbohydrates

Carbohydrates play a pivotal role in sustaining the body's energy needs and promoting overall health.

Here are key reasons highlighting the importance of carbohydrates:

1.   **Primary Energy Source:** Carbohydrates serve as the body's primary and most efficient source of energy. When consumed, they are broken down into glucose, a form of sugar that fuels various bodily functions, including brain activity and muscle contractions.

2.   **Brain Function:** The brain heavily relies on glucose for energy. Adequate carbohydrate intake ensures a steady supply of glucose to the brain, supporting cognitive functions such

as concentration, memory, and decision-making.

3. **Exercise Performance:** Carbohydrates are crucial for athletes and individuals engaged in physical activities. During exercise, the body uses glycogen, the stored form of glucose, for energy. Consuming carbohydrates before and after workouts helps replenish glycogen stores and enhances endurance.

4. **Metabolic Regulation:** Carbohydrates play a role in regulating metabolism. Insulin, a hormone released in response to carbohydrate consumption, helps control blood sugar levels. Balanced carbohydrate intake contributes to stable blood sugar levels, reducing the risk of metabolic disorders.

5.   **Digestive   Health:**   Carbohydrates, particularly dietary fiber found in whole grains, fruits, and vegetables, promote digestive health. Fiber adds bulk to stool, preventing constipation, and supporting a healthy gut microbiome.

6.   **Nutrient Density:** Many carbohydrate-rich foods, such as whole grains, fruits, and legumes, are nutrient-dense, providing essential vitamins, minerals, and antioxidants. Including a variety of these foods in the diet contributes to overall well-being.

7.   **Weight   Management:**   Choosing complex carbohydrates over refined options promotes a feeling of fullness and helps control appetite. This can contribute to weight management by reducing the likelihood of overeating.

Types of Carbohydrates

Understanding the types of carbohydrates is crucial for making informed dietary choices. Opting for complex carbohydrates from whole, unprocessed sources provides sustained energy and essential nutrients, contributing to overall health and well-being.

1. Simple Carbohydrates (Sugars):

- **Monosaccharides:** These are single sugar molecules.

    - *Glucose:* A primary source of energy for cells.

    - *Fructose:* Found in fruits and honey.

    - *Galactose:* Present in milk and dairy products.

- **Disaccharides:** Formed by the combination of two monosaccharides.

- *Sucrose (table sugar):* Glucose + Fructose.

- *Lactose (milk sugar):* Glucose + Galactose.

- *Maltose:* Glucose + Glucose.

2. Complex Carbohydrates (Polysaccharides):

- **Starch:** A complex carbohydrate found in plants, such as grains, legumes, and tubers. It consists of glucose units linked together.

- **Glycogen:** The storage form of glucose in animals, particularly in the liver and muscles. It serves as a quick energy reserve.

- **Fiber:** A type of carbohydrate that the body cannot fully digest.

- *Soluble Fiber:* Dissolves in water and can help lower cholesterol. Found in oats, beans, and fruits.

- *Insoluble Fiber:* Does not dissolve in water and adds bulk to the stool. Found in whole grains, vegetables, and nuts.

3. Dietary Sources:

- **Whole Grains:** Brown rice, oats, quinoa, and whole wheat.

- **Fruits:** Rich in fructose and fiber.

- **Vegetables:** Provide various types of carbohydrates along with fiber and nutrients.

- **Legumes:** Beans, lentils, and chickpeas are excellent sources of complex carbohydrates and fiber.

- **Dairy:** Contains lactose, a disaccharide found in milk.

Chapter 3

Debunking Carb Myths

Carbs are the Enemy

The belief that "carbs are the enemy" oversimplifies the complex role of carbohydrates in nutrition. While it's true that excessive consumption of refined and processed carbohydrates can have adverse effects on health, demonizing all carbs is an overly broad and inaccurate perspective.

Carbohydrates are the body's primary source of energy, crucial for fueling essential bodily functions, including brain activity and muscle function. However, not all carbs are equal. Whole, unprocessed carbohydrates found in fruits, vegetables, and whole grains offer essential nutrients and a slower release of energy. On the other hand, refined carbs, prevalent in sugary snacks and processed foods, lack many nutrients and can lead to rapid spikes in blood sugar levels.

A balanced approach to carbohydrate intake is key. Eliminating entire food groups, including carbohydrates, can result in nutritional deficiencies and an imbalanced diet. Individual nutritional needs vary based on factors like age, activity level, and health status. Choosing complex carbohydrates supports overall health and weight management by promoting feelings of fullness.

All Carbs are Equal

The notion that "all carbs are equal" oversimplifies the diverse nature of carbohydrates and their impact on health. Carbohydrates, as a macronutrient, encompass a wide range of compounds, and their effects on the body vary significantly based on their complexity and source.

Simple carbohydrates, found in sugary snacks and processed foods, provide a quick source of energy but lack essential nutrients. In contrast, complex carbohydrates, prevalent in whole grains, fruits, and vegetables, offer a more sustained release of energy along with vital vitamins, minerals, and fiber.

While it is true that all carbohydrates ultimately break down into glucose, their journey through the digestive system differs. Simple carbs often lead to rapid spikes in blood sugar levels, potentially contributing to energy crashes and cravings. On the other hand, complex carbs, with their fiber content, promote a slower and more controlled release of glucose, providing lasting energy and supporting digestive health.

The blanket statement that "all carbs are equal" ignores the importance of choosing nutrient-dense, whole food sources over refined options. Additionally, individual factors such as metabolism, activity level, and overall health influence how the body processes and utilizes carbohydrates.

Low-carb diets are the Only Solution

The belief that "low-carb diets are the only solution" oversimplifies the complex landscape of nutritional needs and weight management. While low-carb diets have gained popularity for their potential to facilitate weight loss, declaring them as the sole solution disregards the nuanced relationship between carbohydrates and overall health.

Carbohydrates are a primary source of energy for the body, particularly the brain and muscles. Restricting carbohydrates severely may lead to insufficient energy levels, impacting cognitive function and physical performance. While reducing refined and processed carbohydrates is beneficial, eliminating entire food groups can deprive the body of essential nutrients found in whole grains, fruits, and vegetables.

Moreover, the effectiveness of dietary approaches varies among individuals. Factors such as metabolic rate, activity level, and overall health influence the body's response to different diets. What works for one person may not be suitable for another.

Balanced nutrition involves considering the quality of carbohydrates rather than adopting a one-size-fits-all approach. Choosing complex carbohydrates over refined options, emphasizing whole foods, and maintaining an overall balanced diet are essential for sustained well-being.

Chapter 4

The Science Behind Carb Metabolism

How the Body Processes Carbs

The body undergoes a sophisticated process to convert carbohydrates into energy, a crucial mechanism for sustaining various physiological functions. The journey begins with the ingestion of carbohydrates through dietary sources such as grains, fruits, and vegetables.

1. Digestion:

- The process starts in the mouth, where salivary enzymes break down complex carbohydrates into smaller units. Amylase, an enzyme, initiates the breakdown of starches into maltose.

- In the stomach, carbohydrates are further broken down into simpler compounds, setting the stage for absorption in the small intestine.

2. Absorption:

- The majority of carbohydrate absorption occurs in the small intestine. Enzymes, including maltase, sucrase, and lactase, break down disaccharides like maltose, sucrose, and lactose into monosaccharides.

- Glucose, fructose, and galactose, the primary monosaccharides, are then absorbed through the intestinal lining into the bloodstream.

3. Transportation:

- Once in the bloodstream, glucose travels to various cells throughout the body, providing a readily available energy source.

- Insulin, a hormone released by the pancreas, plays a crucial role in facilitating the uptake of glucose by cells. It acts as a "key," allowing cells to absorb glucose for energy.

4. Utilization and Storage:

- Cells use glucose for immediate energy needs. The brain, in particular, heavily relies on glucose for its functioning.

- Excess glucose is stored in the liver and muscles as glycogen, a form of stored energy. This glycogen can be broken down back into glucose when energy demands rise.

5. Energy Production:

- During periods of increased energy demand, such as physical activity, glycogen is converted back into glucose and released into the bloodstream.

- Through a process called glycolysis, glucose is broken down in the cells to produce adenosine triphosphate (ATP), the body's primary energy currency.

6. Metabolic Regulation:

- The body regulates blood sugar levels to maintain a steady supply of energy. Insulin promotes the uptake of glucose when levels are high, while glucagon signals the release of stored glucose when levels drop.

Glycemic Index and Load

The glycemic index (GI) and glycemic load (GL) are important concepts in understanding how different carbohydrates affect blood sugar levels. Here's an overview of these terms and their significance:

Glycemic Index (GI):

The glycemic index measures how quickly a carbohydrate-containing food raises blood sugar levels. It is a numerical scale ranging from 0 to 100, with higher values indicating a faster and more significant increase in blood sugar. The classification is as follows:

- **Low GI (0-55):** Foods that cause a slower, more gradual rise in blood sugar. Examples include most vegetables, legumes, and whole grains.

- **Medium GI (56-69):** Foods with a moderate impact on blood sugar, such as certain fruits and whole wheat products.

- **High GI (70 and above):** Foods that rapidly raise blood sugar levels.

Examples include white bread, sugary cereals, and certain processed snacks.

Factors Influencing Glycemic Index:

Several factors can affect a food's glycemic index, including its fiber content, the presence of fat and protein, and the degree of food processing. Generally, foods with more fiber and those that are less processed tend to have a lower glycemic index.

Glycemic Load (GL):

While the glycemic index provides information about the quality of carbohydrates, the glycemic load considers both quality and quantity. It takes into account not only how quickly a food raises blood sugar but also the actual amount of carbohydrates consumed. The formula for calculating glycemic load is:

Glycemic Load=(GI×Carbohydrate content (
g)100)Glycemic Load=(100GI×Carbohydrate
content (g))

- **Low GL (0-10):** Foods with a minimal impact on blood sugar.

- **Medium GL (11-19):** Foods with a moderate impact.

- **High GL (20 and above):** Foods that can lead to a significant increase in blood sugar.

Significance:

- **Blood Sugar Control:** Understanding the glycemic index and load can help individuals manage blood sugar levels, which is crucial for those with diabetes or those aiming for sustained energy levels.

- **Weight Management:** Choosing foods with a lower glycemic load may aid in weight management by promoting a more stable and gradual release of energy, reducing the likelihood of overeating.

Chapter 5

Carb Confusion and Weight Management

Understanding the Link

Carb confusion often arises in discussions about weight management, leading to misconceptions about the role of carbohydrates in achieving and maintaining a healthy weight. Understanding the link between carbohydrate consumption and weight management is crucial for making informed dietary choices.

Carbohydrates, as a primary source of energy, play a significant role in the body's metabolism. However, not all carbs are created equal, and it's the quality of carbohydrates that matters most. Highly processed and refined carbohydrates, often found in sugary snacks and white bread, can contribute to weight gain due to their rapid impact on blood sugar levels and the potential for overeating.

Choosing complex carbohydrates, such as whole grains, fruits, and vegetables, supports weight management. These foods are rich in fiber, promoting a feeling of fullness and reducing overall calorie intake. Additionally, they provide essential nutrients, contributing to overall well-being.

The confusion often arises from extreme approaches, such as overly restrictive low-carb diets. While reducing intake of refined carbs can be beneficial, complete elimination is unnecessary and may lead to nutritional imbalances.

Balancing carbohydrate intake with proteins and healthy fats is a key aspect of sustainable weight management. It prevents the energy crashes associated with excessive refined carbs and supports a steady release of energy throughout the day.

Finding Your Carb Balance

This is a personalized journey that involves understanding your body's unique response to carbohydrates and tailoring your intake to meet your health and fitness goals.

Here are key steps to help you find the right carb balance for you:

1. **Assess Your Goals:** Clearly define your health and fitness objectives. Whether it's weight management, improved energy levels, or specific athletic performance, your goals will influence your ideal carb balance.

2. **Understand Your Body:** Pay attention to how your body responds to different

types and amounts of carbohydrates. Note your energy levels, mood, and performance after consuming meals with varying carb content.

3. **Differentiate Between Carbs:** Recognize the distinction between simple and complex carbohydrates. Choose complex carbs from whole, unprocessed sources like whole grains, fruits, and vegetables, as they provide sustained energy and essential nutrients.

4. **Consider Your Activity Level:** Adjust your carb intake based on your activity level. Those engaged in regular physical activity may require more carbohydrates to support energy needs, especially around workout times.

5. **Listen to Hunger and Fullness Cues:** Pay attention to your body's hunger and

fullness signals. Eating mindfully can help you determine when and how much to eat, preventing overconsumption of carbs.

6. **Monitor Blood Sugar Levels:** For individuals with diabetes or those concerned about blood sugar regulation, monitoring blood sugar levels can provide insights into how different foods impact your body.

7. **Consult with a Professional:** If you have specific health concerns or dietary goals, consider consulting with a healthcare professional or a registered dietitian. They can provide personalized guidance based on your individual needs.

8. **Experiment and Adjust:** Finding your carb balance may involve some trial

and error. Experiment with different carbohydrate ratios, types, and timing, and observe how your body responds. Adjust your approach based on what works best for you.

Chapter 6

Healthy Carbohydrate Food Sources

A healthy diet includes a variety of nutrient-dense carbohydrates that provide essential energy, fiber, vitamins, and minerals.

Here are list of healthy carbohydrate food sources:

Whole Grains:

1. Quinoa: A complete protein source with high fiber content.

2. Brown Rice: Rich in fiber, B vitamins, and minerals.

3. Oats: High in soluble fiber and beta-glucans for heart health.

4. Barley: Contains both soluble and insoluble fiber, supporting digestion.

5. Buckwheat: Gluten-free and a good source of protein and antioxidants.

6. Farro: High in fiber, protein, and nutrients like magnesium and zinc.

7. Millet: Packed with essential amino acids, vitamins, and minerals.

8. Amaranth: Gluten-free and rich in protein, fiber, and micronutrients.

Legumes:

1. Lentils: High in protein, fiber, and various vitamins and minerals.

2. Chickpeas: Good source of protein, fiber, and folate.

3. Black Beans: Rich in fiber, protein, and antioxidants.

4. Kidney Beans: Provide protein, fiber, and essential minerals.

5. Edamame: Young soybeans rich in protein, fiber, and vitamins.

6. Split Peas: High in fiber, protein, and folate.

Fruits:

1. Berries (Blueberries, Strawberries, Raspberries): Packed with antioxidants, vitamins, and fiber.

2. Apples: Provide fiber, vitamins, and antioxidants.

3. Bananas: Rich in potassium, vitamins, and natural sugars.

4. Oranges: High in vitamin C, fiber, and various antioxidants.

5. Pears: Contain dietary fiber, vitamins, and minerals.

Vegetables:

1. Sweet Potatoes: Excellent source of complex carbs, fiber, and beta-carotene.

2. Broccoli: Low in calories, high in fiber, vitamins, and antioxidants.

3. Spinach: Low-calorie leafy green rich in vitamins and minerals.

4. Carrots: Provide beta-carotene, fiber, and vitamins.

5. Brussels Sprouts: High in fiber, vitamins, and antioxidants.

Whole Grain Products:

1. Whole Wheat Bread: Contains fiber, B vitamins, and minerals.

2. Whole Grain Pasta: Rich in fiber and nutrients.

3. Quinoa Pasta: Gluten-free alternative with protein and fiber.

4. Brown Rice Cakes: Low-calorie snack with complex carbs.

Nuts and Seeds:

1. Chia Seeds: Packed with fiber, omega-3 fatty acids, and antioxidants.

2. Flaxseeds: High in fiber, omega-3s, and lignans.

3. Oats (Oatmeal): Whole grain goodness with fiber and nutrients.

4. Almonds: Provide healthy fats, protein, and fiber.

Chapter 8

Meal Plans for Carb Clarity

Week 1

Day 1:

- **Breakfast:** Scrambled eggs with spinach and whole grain toast.

- **Snack:** Greek yogurt with a handful of mixed berries.

- **Lunch:** Quinoa salad with mixed vegetables and grilled chicken.

- **Dessert:** Dark chocolate-covered strawberries.

- **Dinner:** Baked salmon with sweet potato and steamed broccoli.

Day 2:

- **Breakfast:** Whole grain English muffin with avocado and poached eggs.

- **Snack:** Apple slices with almond butter.

- **Lunch:** Lentil soup with a side of whole grain crackers.

- **Dessert:** Chia seed pudding with vanilla and berries.

- **Dinner:** Stir-fried tofu with brown rice and a variety of colorful vegetables.

Day 3:

- **Breakfast:** Oatmeal with sliced bananas and a drizzle of honey.

- **Snack:** Cottage cheese with pineapple chunks.

- **Lunch:** Chickpea salad with cucumber, cherry tomatoes, and feta cheese.

- **Dessert:** Frozen yogurt with mixed berries.

- **Dinner:** Turkey chili with black beans, served over quinoa.

Day 4:

- **Breakfast:** Smoothie with kale, pineapple, Greek yogurt, and a touch of almond butter.

- **Snack:** Hummus with carrot and cucumber sticks.

- **Lunch:** Whole wheat wrap with grilled chicken, hummus, and veggies.

- **Dessert:** Baked apple slices with cinnamon.

- **Dinner:** Shrimp stir-fry with broccoli, bell peppers, and brown rice.

Day 5:

- **Breakfast:** Greek yogurt parfait with granola and mixed berries.

- **Snack:** Mixed nuts and dried fruits.

- **Lunch:** Quinoa and black bean bowl with salsa and avocado.

- **Dessert:** Dark chocolate-covered almonds.

- **Dinner:** Baked chicken breast with quinoa and roasted Brussels sprouts.

Day 6:

- **Breakfast:** Banana and walnut muffins made with whole grain flour.

- **Snack:** Sliced cucumber with tzatziki.

- **Lunch:** Spinach and feta-stuffed chicken breast with a side of roasted sweet potatoes.

- **Dessert:** Coconut milk rice pudding.

- **Dinner:** Vegetable curry with lentils served over brown rice.

Day 7:

- **Breakfast:** Whole grain pancakes with blueberries and a dollop of Greek yogurt.

- **Snack:** Fresh fruit salad.

- **Lunch:** Caprese salad with whole grain croutons and grilled chicken.

- **Dessert:** Berry and yogurt parfait.

- **Dinner:** Beef and vegetable kebabs with quinoa.

Week 2

Day 8:

- **Breakfast:** Overnight oats with almond milk, topped with sliced peaches.

- **Snack:** Cottage cheese with a drizzle of honey.

- **Lunch:** Turkey and avocado lettuce wraps with cherry tomatoes.

- **Dessert:** Dark chocolate-covered banana slices.

- **Dinner:** Grilled fish tacos with whole wheat tortillas and a cabbage slaw.

Day 9:

- **Breakfast:** Whole grain bagel with smoked salmon, cream cheese, and capers.

- **Snack:** Mixed berries with a dollop of whipped cream.

- **Lunch:** Lentil and vegetable curry served over cauliflower rice.

- **Dessert:** Frozen mango yogurt bites.

- **Dinner:** Baked chicken thighs with quinoa and roasted asparagus.

Day 10:

- **Breakfast:** Smoothie bowl with spinach, banana, and a sprinkle of granola.

- **Snack:** Greek yogurt with mixed nuts.

- **Lunch:** Caprese quinoa salad with balsamic vinaigrette.

- **Dessert:** Raspberry chia seed pudding.

- **Dinner:** Stir-fried tempeh with broccoli and brown rice.

Day 11:

- **Breakfast:** Whole grain waffles with fresh berries and a drizzle of maple syrup.

- **Snack:** Edamame with sea salt.

- **Lunch:** Chicken Caesar salad with whole grain croutons.

- **Dessert:** Baked pear with cinnamon.

- **Dinner:** Grilled shrimp skewers with quinoa and sautéed zucchini.

Day 12:

- **Breakfast:** Avocado and tomato omelet with a side of whole grain toast.

- **Snack:** Cherry tomato and mozzarella skewers.

- **Lunch:** Mediterranean quinoa bowl with olives and feta.

- **Dessert:** Almond and coconut energy balls.

- **Dinner:** Beef and broccoli stir-fry with brown rice.

Day 13:

- **Breakfast:** Peanut butter and banana smoothie.

- **Snack:** Carrot and cucumber sticks with hummus.

- **Lunch:** Spinach and feta-stuffed portobello mushrooms with a side salad.

- **Dessert:** Mango sorbet.

- **Dinner:** Spaghetti squash with turkey meatballs and marinara sauce.

Day 14:

- **Breakfast:** Whole grain toast with smashed avocado and poached eggs.

- **Snack:** Sliced apples with a sprinkle of cinnamon.

- **Lunch:** Quinoa-stuffed bell peppers with black beans and corn.

- **Dessert:** Dark chocolate-dipped strawberries.

- **Dinner:** Baked cod with a quinoa and mixed vegetable medley.

Chapter 10

Breakfast Recipes for Balanced Carb Meals

Oatmeal with Nut Butter and Banana:

Ingredients:

- 1/2 cup rolled oats

- 1 cup almond milk

- 1 tablespoon almond or peanut butter

- 1 banana, sliced

- 1 teaspoon chia seeds

Instructions:

1. Cook oats in almond milk until creamy.
2. Top with nut butter, banana slices, and chia seeds.

Nutritional Information:

- Calories: 350

- Protein: 10g

- Fat: 15g

- Carbohydrates: 45g

- Fiber: 8g

Greek Yogurt Parfait:

Ingredients:

- 1 cup Greek yogurt

- 1/2 cup granola

- 1/2 cup mixed berries

- 1 tablespoon honey

Instructions:

1. Layer Greek yogurt with granola and berries.

2. Drizzle with honey.

Nutritional Information:

- Calories: 300

- Protein: 20g

- Fat: 8g

- Carbohydrates: 40g

- Fiber: 6g

Vegetable Omelet with Whole Grain Toast:

Ingredients:

- 2 eggs

- Assorted vegetables (spinach, bell peppers, tomatoes)

- 1 slice whole grain bread

Instructions:

1. Whisk eggs and cook with vegetables.

2. Serve with a slice of whole-grain toast.

Nutritional Information:

- Calories: 250

- Protein: 15g

- Fat: 12g

- Carbohydrates: 20g

- Fiber: 4g

Quinoa Breakfast Bowl:

Ingredients:

- 1/2 cup cooked quinoa

- 1/2 cup almond milk

- Sliced fruits (strawberries, kiwi)

- 2 tablespoons chopped nuts

Instructions:

1. Mix quinoa with almond milk.

2. Top with sliced fruits and chopped nuts.

Nutritional Information:

- Calories: 300

- Protein: 8g

- Fat: 12g

- Carbohydrates: 40g

- Fiber: 6g

Avocado and Smoked Salmon Bagel:

Ingredients:

- 1 whole grain bagel

- 1/2 avocado, mashed

- 2 ounces smoked salmon

- Chopped chives for garnish

Instructions:

1. Spread mashed avocado on the bagel.

2.   Top with smoked salmon and garnish with chives.

Nutritional Information:

- Calories: 380

- Protein: 20g

- Fat: 15g

- Carbohydrates: 40g

- Fiber: 8g

Whole Wheat Pancakes with Berries:

Ingredients:

- 1 cup whole wheat flour

- 1 tablespoon honey

- 1 teaspoon baking powder

- 1 cup almond milk

- Mixed berries for topping

Instructions:

1. Mix ingredients to make pancake batter.
2. Cook pancakes and top with mixed berries.

Nutritional Information:

- Calories: 320
- Protein: 10g
- Fat: 5g
- Carbohydrates: 60g
- Fiber: 8g

Smoothie Bowl:

Ingredients:

- 1 cup spinach
- 1 banana
- 1/2 cup Greek yogurt
- 1/2 cup almond milk

- Granola, chia seeds, and sliced almonds for topping

Instructions:

1. Blend spinach, banana, yogurt, and almond milk.

2. Pour into a bowl and top with granola, chia seeds, and sliced almonds.

Nutritional Information:

- Calories: 280

- Protein: 15g

- Fat: 10g

- Carbohydrates: 35g

- Fiber: 7g

Sweet Potato and Black Bean Breakfast Burrito:

Ingredients:

- 1 whole wheat tortilla

- Scrambled eggs

- Cooked sweet potatoes

- Black beans

- Salsa for topping

Instructions:

1. Fill the tortilla with scrambled eggs, sweet potatoes, and black beans.

2. Top with salsa.

Nutritional Information:

- Calories: 340

- Protein: 15g

- Fat: 10g

- Carbohydrates: 45g

- Fiber: 10g

Fruit and Nut Overnight Oats:

Ingredients:

- 1/2 cup rolled oats

- 1/2 cup almond milk

- Mixed fruits (berries, mango)

- 2 tablespoons mixed nuts

- **Instructions:**

1. Mix oats with almond milk and refrigerate overnight.

2. Top with mixed fruits and nuts.

- **Nutritional Information:**

- Calories: 280

- Protein: 8g

- Fat: 12g

- Carbohydrates: 35g

- Fiber: 6g

Egg and Veggie Breakfast Muffins:

Ingredients:

- 4 eggs

- Diced vegetables (bell peppers, spinach)

- 1/4 cup shredded cheese

Instructions:

1. Whisk eggs and mix with diced vegetables.

2. Pour into muffin tins, sprinkle with cheese, and bake.

Nutritional Information:

- Calories: 220

- Protein: 15g

- Fat: 14g

- Carbohydrates: 8g

- Fiber: 2g

Chapter 11

Lunch Recipes for Balanced Carb Meals

Quinoa and Black Bean Salad:

Ingredients:

- 1 cup cooked quinoa

- 1/2 cup black beans (canned, drained)

- Cherry tomatoes, diced

- Cucumber, diced

- Feta cheese, crumbled

- Olive oil, lemon juice, salt, and pepper for dressing

Instructions:

1. Combine quinoa, black beans, tomatoes, cucumber, and feta.

2. Whisk olive oil, lemon juice, salt, and pepper for dressing.

3. Toss salad with dressing.

Nutritional Information:

- Calories: 400

- Protein: 15g

- Fat: 15g

- Carbohydrates: 55g

- Fiber: 10g

Grilled Chicken and Vegetable Wrap:

Ingredients:

- Grilled chicken breast

- Whole wheat wrap

- Mixed vegetables (bell peppers, onions, zucchini)

- Hummus for spreading

Instructions:

1. Grill chicken and vegetables.
2. Fill the wrap with chicken, veggies, and hummus.

Nutritional Information:

- Calories: 380

- Protein: 25g

- Fat: 10g

- Carbohydrates: 45g

- Fiber: 8g

Salmon and Quinoa Bowl:

Ingredients:

- Baked or grilled salmon

- 1 cup cooked quinoa

- Steamed broccoli

- Avocado slices

- Soy sauce or teriyaki sauce for drizzling

Instructions:

1. Place quinoa in a bowl, and top with salmon, broccoli, and avocado.
2. Drizzle with soy sauce or teriyaki sauce.

Nutritional Information:

- Calories: 420

- Protein: 30g

- Fat: 20g

- Carbohydrates: 35g

- Fiber: 8g

Mediterranean Chickpea Salad:

Ingredients:

- 1 can chickpeas (canned, drained)

- Cherry tomatoes, halved

- Cucumber, diced

- Kalamata olives, sliced

- Feta cheese, crumbled

- Olive oil, balsamic vinegar, salt, and pepper for dressing

Instructions:

1. Combine chickpeas, tomatoes, cucumber, olives, and feta.

2. Whisk olive oil, balsamic vinegar, salt, and pepper for dressing.

3. Toss salad with dressing.

Nutritional Information:

- Calories: 380

- Protein: 15g

- Fat: 18g

- Carbohydrates: 40g

- Fiber: 12g

Turkey and Vegetable Stir-Fry:

Ingredients:

- Ground turkey

- Mixed vegetables (broccoli, bell peppers, snap peas)

- Brown rice

- Soy sauce, ginger, and garlic for seasoning

Instructions:

1. Cook ground turkey and stir-fry with vegetables.
2. Season with soy sauce, ginger, and garlic.
3. Serve over brown rice.

Nutritional Information:

- Calories: 420

- Protein: 25g

- Fat: 10g

- Carbohydrates: 55g

- Fiber: 8g

Caprese Quinoa Bowl:

Ingredients:

- 1 cup cooked quinoa

- Cherry tomatoes, halved

- Fresh mozzarella, diced

- Fresh basil leaves

- Balsamic glaze for drizzling

Instructions:

1. Combine quinoa, tomatoes, mozzarella, and basil.
2. Drizzle with balsamic glaze.

Nutritional Information:

- Calories: 350

- Protein: 15g

- Fat: 18g

- Carbohydrates: 35g

- Fiber: 6g

Shrimp and Vegetable Whole Wheat Pasta:

Ingredients:

- Whole wheat pasta
- Shrimp, peeled and deveined
- Mixed vegetables (bell peppers, cherry tomatoes, spinach)
- Olive oil, garlic, and red pepper flakes for seasoning

Instructions:

1. Cook pasta and sauté shrimp with vegetables.
2. Season with olive oil, garlic, and red pepper flakes.

Nutritional Information:

- Calories: 420
- Protein: 20g

- Fat: 15g

- Carbohydrates: 55g

- Fiber: 10g

Chickpea and Spinach Stuffed Sweet Potatoes:

Ingredients:

- Sweet potatoes, baked

- Chickpeas, canned and drained

- Spinach, sautéed

- Greek yogurt for topping

Instructions:

1. Split baked sweet potatoes and fill with chickpeas and sautéed spinach.
2. Top with Greek yogurt.

Nutritional Information:

- Calories: 380

- Protein: 15g

- Fat: 8g

- Carbohydrates: 65g

- Fiber: 12g

Vegetarian Burrito Bowl:

Ingredients:

- Black beans, cooked

- Brown rice

- Corn, cooked

- Avocado slices

- Salsa and cilantro for topping

Instructions:

1. Combine black beans, brown rice, corn, and avocado.

2. Top with salsa and cilantro.

Nutritional Information:

- Calories: 400

- Protein: 15g

- Fat: 12g

- Carbohydrates: 60g

- Fiber: 14g

Egg and Vegetable Quiche:

Ingredients:

- Whole wheat pie crust

- Eggs

- Mixed vegetables (bell peppers, onions, spinach)

- Feta cheese, crumbled

Instructions:

1. Whisk eggs and mix with sautéed vegetables and feta.
2. Pour into the pie crust and bake until set.

Nutritional Information:

- Calories: 350
- Protein: 15g
- Fat: 18g
- Carbohydrates: 30g
- Fiber: 6g

Chapter 12

Dinner Recipes for Balanced Carb Meals

Grilled Chicken Quinoa Bowl:

Ingredients:

- Grilled chicken breast

- 1 cup cooked quinoa

- Roasted vegetables (zucchini, cherry tomatoes, bell peppers)

- Olive oil, lemon juice, salt, and pepper for seasoning

Instructions:

1. Grill chicken and roast vegetables.
2. Serve over cooked quinoa.
3. Drizzle with olive oil, lemon juice, salt, and pepper.

Nutritional Information:

- Calories: 450

- Protein: 35g

- Fat: 15g

- Carbohydrates: 45g

- Fiber: 8g

Salmon and Asparagus Foil Packets:

Ingredients:

- Salmon fillets

- Asparagus spears

- Lemon slices

- Garlic, minced

- Olive oil, salt, and pepper

Instructions:

1. Place salmon, asparagus, and lemon slices on foil.
2. Sprinkle with minced garlic, olive oil, salt, and pepper.
3. Seal and bake in foil packets.

Nutritional Information:

- Calories: 380
- Protein: 30g
- Fat: 20g
- Carbohydrates: 10g
- Fiber: 5g

Vegetarian Stir-Fry with Tofu:

Ingredients:

- Extra-firm tofu, cubed

- Mixed vegetables (broccoli, bell peppers, snap peas)

- Brown rice

- Soy sauce, ginger, and garlic for seasoning

Instructions:

1. Sauté tofu and vegetables.
2. Season with soy sauce, ginger, and garlic.
3. Serve over brown rice.

Nutritional Information:

- Calories: 420

- Protein: 20g

- Fat: 15g

- Carbohydrates: 55g

- Fiber: 8g

Baked Chicken Parmesan:

Ingredients:

- Chicken breasts pounded thin
- Whole wheat breadcrumbs
- Marinara sauce
- Mozzarella cheese, shredded
- Parmesan cheese, grated

Instructions:

1. Coat chicken in breadcrumbs and bake.
2. Top with marinara sauce and cheese.
3. Bake until the cheese is melted.

Nutritional Information:

- Calories: 380
- Protein: 35g
- Fat: 12g

- Carbohydrates: 30g

- Fiber: 5g

Shrimp and Vegetable Stir-Fried Noodles:

Ingredients:

- Whole wheat noodles

- Shrimp, peeled and deveined

- Mixed vegetables (bell peppers, broccoli, carrots)

- Soy sauce, sesame oil, and ginger for seasoning

Instructions:

1. Cook noodles and stir-fry shrimp and vegetables.
2. Season with soy sauce, sesame oil, and ginger.

Nutritional Information:

- Calories: 400

- Protein: 25g

- Fat: 10g

- Carbohydrates: 55g

- Fiber: 8g

Vegetarian Lentil Soup:

Ingredients:

- Lentils rinsed

- Mixed vegetables (carrots, celery, onions)

- Vegetable broth

- Tomato sauce

- Garlic and herbs for seasoning

Instructions:

1. Cook lentils and vegetables in vegetable broth.

2. Add tomato sauce and season with garlic and herbs.

Nutritional Information:

- Calories: 350

- Protein: 18g

- Fat: 2g

- Carbohydrates: 60g

- Fiber: 15g

Turkey and Quinoa Stuffed Peppers:

Ingredients:

- Ground turkey

- Quinoa, cooked

- Bell peppers, halved

- Tomato sauce

- Italian seasoning, salt, and pepper

Instructions:

1. Cook ground turkey and quinoa.
2. Mix with tomato sauce and seasonings.
3. Stuff peppers and bake until tender.

Nutritional Information:

- Calories: 380

- Protein: 25g

- Fat: 10g

- Carbohydrates: 45g

- Fiber: 8g

Vegetable and Chickpea Curry:

Ingredients:

- Chickpeas, canned and drained

- Mixed vegetables (cauliflower, peas, carrots)

- Coconut milk

- Curry powder, cumin, and coriander for seasoning

Instructions:

1. Cook chickpeas and vegetables in coconut milk.
2. Season with curry powder, cumin, and coriander.

Nutritional Information:

- Calories: 420

- Protein: 15g

- Fat: 18g

- Carbohydrates: 55g

- Fiber: 12g

Baked Cod with Sweet Potato Wedges:

Ingredients:

- Cod fillets

- Sweet potatoes, cut into wedges

- Olive oil, paprika, and garlic powder for seasoning

Instructions:

1. Season cod with olive oil, paprika, and garlic powder.
2. Bake cod and sweet potato wedges until cooked.

Nutritional Information:

- Calories: 350

- Protein: 30g

- Fat: 10g

- Carbohydrates: 35g

- Fiber: 6g

Mushroom and Spinach Stuffed Chicken Breast:

Ingredients:

- Chicken breasts

- Mushrooms, chopped

- Spinach wilted

- Mozzarella cheese, shredded

Instructions:

1. Stuff chicken with mushrooms, spinach, and cheese.
2. Bake until chicken is cooked through.

Nutritional Information:

- Calories: 380

- Protein: 40g

- Fat: 15g

- Carbohydrates: 25g

- Fiber: 5g

Chapter 13

Snack Recipes for Balanced Carb Meals

Greek Yogurt and Berry Parfait:

Ingredients:

- Greek yogurt

- Mixed berries (strawberries, blueberries, raspberries)

- Granola

- Honey

Instructions:

1. Layer Greek yogurt with mixed berries.
2. Top with granola and drizzle with honey.

Nutritional Information:

- Calories: 200

- Protein: 15g

- Fat: 5g

- Carbohydrates: 30g

- Fiber: 5g

Apple Slices with Almond Butter:

Ingredients:

- Apple, sliced

- Almond butter

Instructions:

1. Spread almond butter on apple slices.

Nutritional Information:

- Calories: 180

- Protein: 4g

- Fat: 10g

- Carbohydrates: 20g

- Fiber: 5g

Trail Mix with Nuts and Dried Fruit:

Ingredients:

- Mixed nuts (almonds, walnuts, cashews)

- Dried fruits (raisins, cranberries)

- Dark chocolate chips

Instructions:

- Mix nuts, dried fruits, and dark chocolate chips.

Nutritional Information:

- Calories: 250

- Protein: 7g

- Fat: 15g

- Carbohydrates: 25g

- Fiber: 4g

Whole Grain Crackers with Hummus:

Ingredients:

- Whole grain crackers

- Hummus

Instructions:

- Spread hummus on whole-grain crackers.

Nutritional Information:

- Calories: 180

- Protein: 6g

- Fat: 8g

- Carbohydrates: 20g

- Fiber: 4g

Cottage Cheese with Pineapple:

Ingredients:

- Cottage cheese

- Pineapple chunks

Instructions:

- Mix cottage cheese with pineapple chunks.

Nutritional Information:

- Calories: 150

- Protein: 15g

- Fat: 2g

- Carbohydrates: 20g

- Fiber: 2g

Vegetable Sticks with Hummus:

Ingredients:

- Carrot sticks

- Celery sticks

- Bell pepper strips

- Hummus

Instructions:

- Dip vegetable sticks in hummus.

Nutritional Information:

- Calories: 100

- Protein: 3g

- Fat: 5g

- Carbohydrates: 15g

- Fiber: 5g

Cheese and Whole Grain Crackers:

Ingredients:

- Cheese slices or cubes

- Whole grain crackers

Instructions:

- Pair cheese with whole-grain crackers.

Nutritional Information:

- Calories: 220

- Protein: 10g

- Fat: 15g

- Carbohydrates: 15g

- Fiber: 3g

Yogurt-Dipped Strawberries:

Ingredients:

- Strawberries

- Greek yogurt

- Honey

Instructions:

- Dip strawberries in Greek yogurt.
- Drizzle with honey.

Nutritional Information:

- Calories: 160

- Protein: 8g

- Fat: 5g

- Carbohydrates: 20g

- Fiber: 3g

Hard-Boiled Eggs with Cherry Tomatoes:

Ingredients:

- Hard-boiled eggs

- Cherry tomatoes

Instructions:

- Pair hard-boiled eggs with cherry tomatoes.

Nutritional Information:

- Calories: 140

- Protein: 12g

- Fat: 9g

- Carbohydrates: 4g

- Fiber: 1g

Peanut Butter and Banana Rice Cakes:

Ingredients:

- Rice cakes

- Peanut butter

- Banana slices

Instructions:

1. Spread peanut butter on rice cakes.
2. Top with banana slices.

Nutritional Information:

- Calories: 220

- Protein: 6g

- Fat: 10g

- Carbohydrates: 30g

- Fiber: 4g

Chapter 14

Conclusion

In conclusion, embracing a balanced approach to carbohydrate consumption is the key to unlocking a healthier and more sustainable lifestyle. Throughout this guide, we've explored the intricacies of carbohydrates, debunked common misconceptions, and provided practical insights into making informed choices.

Understanding that not all carbs are created equal empowers you to make conscious decisions about the foods you consume. By appreciating the importance of carbohydrates as a vital energy source for the body, you can build a diet that supports your overall well-being.

Contrary to the notion that carbs are the enemy, we've highlighted the significance of finding your carb balance. It's not about exclusion but about mindful inclusion, ensuring that your diet is rich in nutrient-dense, whole-food sources.

The journey to end carb confusion involves recognizing the diversity of carbohydrates, from complex to simple, and appreciating their unique roles in supporting your health goals. By dispelling the myth that low-carb diets are the only solution, we encourage you to embrace a holistic perspective that aligns with your individual needs and preferences.

Understanding how the body processes carbs, including insights into the glycemic index and load, provides valuable knowledge for making informed dietary choices. By finding your carb balance, you can establish a sustainable eating pattern that promotes not only weight management but also overall health.

To guide you on this journey, we've crafted a 14-day meal plan that incorporates a variety of balanced carb meals, ensuring you enjoy a diverse and satisfying array of flavors. From breakfast to dinner, these recipes are designed to make your culinary experience both enjoyable and health-focused.

Remember, carb confusion is dispelled through education, moderation, and a thoughtful approach to your dietary choices. By implementing the principles outlined in this guide, you are equipped with the tools to navigate the complex world of carbohydrates, empowering you to make choices that align with your health and wellness goals.

As you embark on this journey to end your carb confusion, may you discover the joy of a balanced and nourishing lifestyle, where carbohydrates are not adversaries but allies in

your quest for sustained vitality and well-being.
Cheers to the end of carb confusion and the
beginning of a healthier, happier you!

www.ingramcontent.com/pod-product-compliance
Lightning Source LLC
Chambersburg PA
CBHW071607270726
48661CB00019B/1616